Autism Awareness

How to Recognize the Early Signs and Symptoms in Our Kids

Frank Denver

ISBN: 9781729061558

DEDICATION

To all Lovely Parent who have Autism kids,

look and care for them with your Heart as your Eyes might miss

Something …...

CONTENTS

INTRODUCTION

Autism can be a devastating diagnosis for a parent to receive about their child. There can be a tendency to think that your life will never be the same and the future looks bleak.

This does not have to be the case. Children with autism will require care and special attention, but they will also bring amazing experiences to your life.

There is a saying in the medical world that states "If you know a child with autism, you know one child with autism." No two people with ASD are the same and the sooner you realize your child needs help, the more effective the help will be.

This book will help you take the right steps for your child and provide support for both of you.

CHAPTER 1

UNDERSTANDING AUTISM AND HOW TO DIAGNOSE EARLY

It is important to detect early signs of autism spectrum disorder in infants in order to avoid strained social interactions. If the disorder can be diagnosed before preschool age more can be done to help the child as they begin to interact with other children.

What are the signs of autism in babies?

While every child with autism will display symptoms that are unique to them there are a number of key traits that can act as red flags for a parent to spot potential autism in babies. Autistic babies generally fail to engage with their caretakers in the same way as other infants do and this will manifest in the following ways.

- Non-responsive: Typically, babies respond to gestures by others such as waving and wiggling fingers in front of their face. Cooing and singing should also elicit a response. Autistic babies will often fail to respond to simple stimuli.

- Lack of eye contact: When nursing neurotypical babies will make eye contact with the mother. If there is no eye contact this can indicate an autistic disorder.

- Failure to giggle or smile when engaging with others.

- Clothing and bedding can be distressing for an autistic baby, new materials and textures can lead to the child becoming upset.

- Toys that have loud noises or flashing lights will often cause distress in autistic infants.

- Blank stares when interacting with a caregiver.

- Distress when encountering laughter. Neurotypical babies tend to respond to laughter with their own laughing if your baby is upset by your laughter this could be a sign of autism.

- At the age of 6 months most babies will respond to the sound of their own name by babbling, autistic children will not.

What are the signs of autism in toddlers?

Toddlers with autism will often exhibit the symptoms expressed in infants but can also be expressed via tantrums and temper outbursts. Of course, neurotypical toddlers also have tantrums at this age, but that is more about a power struggle and establishing boundaries. Autistic toddlers will express their very real frustrations with an outburst. The lack of the ability to communicate successfully will often lead to violent tantrums that can be distressing to both the child and the caregiver.

It is also worth noting that autism will manifest itself differently in toddler boys than it will with toddler girls. Below is a list of symptoms that could signal autism in boys and girls.

Early signs of autism in toddler boys.

- Poor social skills: Neurotypical children pick up social skills from their peers and apply them to their own behavior. Autistic boys will commonly display the following behavior.

  Turns their back on others frequently.

  Fails to hug or touch other children or adults.

  Uses other people to function without social interaction. For instance, if a toddler boy leads an adult to the refrigerator when requiring a snack or drink and fails to acknowledge the adults face. Failure to smile or even nod briefly is a common symptom of autism.

- Emotions and communications: Failure to communicate with others even with gestures or sounds.

  When speaking autistic toddlers will often forget the names of their peers and family.

- Restricted interests.

- Sensory issues: This can manifest in two different ways. The toddler will either react to a stimulus in an exaggerated way or will not be unresponsive. It is important to realize that seemingly minor changes to their environment will cause distress in an autistic toddler. Heat and cold can trigger extreme responses and anxiety as can food texture and color.

- Clumsiness and bumping into things. Toddler boys with autism have difficulty knowing where their own bodies are in their personal space. When overwhelmed by their surroundings they can often "not see" people and furniture around them.

Toddler boys have greater difficulty connecting with their caretakers, which can be a major red flag for autism. As such they are more likely to be diagnosed earlier than female toddlers.

What are the signs of autism in female toddlers?

Research shows that only one in three children diagnosed with autism is female. High functioning autism or Asperger's figures show a greater anomaly with only one in nine children being female. This does not necessarily mean that autism is more prevalent in female children, it does mean that misdiagnosis is more common among girls.

Females with autism will display the classically male symptoms but will also display heightened difficulties in social situations. Females have also been known to become intensely aggravated by sensory triggers and are more likely to self-harm.

When do I ask my child's doctor about autism?

Your scheduled checkups will involve your pediatrician assessing your child's progress at regular intervals. However, you may feel that during periods between appointments you have noticed some of the symptoms listed above. You are the person who spends the most time with your child and it is you who may notice that your child is not developing at the same rate as others.

Maybe you feel your child is not engaging with you in the way you expected. Ask your pediatrician to run a series of tests and diagnostic exams. These are non-invasive and will and will include a more detailed assessment of your child. You will also be required to fill in details of your interactions along with any other caregivers.

If you do have concerns, then you may find it useful to make a timeline of symptoms for your pediatrician. Documenting instances of symptoms persistency and frequency will give your pediatrician a clearer view of your child's development. Never be reticent about bringing to attention your concerns about your child. Remember you are the voice of your infant and if your child is autistic an early diagnosis can serve as a platform for early therapies to be applied.

If you feel your doctor is unsure about the diagnosis, then seek a second opinion. The first three years of your child's development are the most important and this is the period when they are the most malleable. If you can implement programs and strategies from an early age the better the prognosis for your child..

CHAPTER 2

TIPS TO HELP A CHILD WITH AUTISM THRIVE

If you have recently learned that your child has or may have autism spectrum disorder you can feel that you have been handed a lifelong battle without any hope of improvement. While it is true that ASD will affect your child for the rest of its life there are treatments that can help the condition become more manageable.

With the correct treatment plan, it is possible to help children develop skills and overcome their development issues. There are multiple services available to help your child and assistance is available at home and through school-based programs to meet your child's personal needs. With the right treatment coupled with love and support your child can learn, thrive and achieve personal growth.

First and foremost, for caregivers of autistic children is the recognition that help is not just available for the child. As a caregiver, it is essential that you stay emotionally strong and look after your own needs as well as your child's. Take help when it is offered and avoid becoming stressed out and unable to cope. This helps nobody, stay strong and emotionally balanced for everyone's sake.

What to do when your child has autism

- Educate yourself: Learn everything you can about the condition and treatments available for ASD children. Take an active part in any discussions about treatments and use your knowledge of your child to ensure the correct treatments are in place.

- Become the voice of your child: ASD children cannot tell the world what they need so that is now your job. Get to know everything you can about your child and use it to help others tailor the treatments they receive. It is important you know the triggers to your child's behaviors

  What makes them happy, what do they enjoy?

What makes them stressed or fearful?

What calms them when they are having a meltdown?

- Celebrate the quirks: Parents often focus on the fact their autistic child is different from other kids and worry about it. Practice acceptance and enjoy the special qualities your child has. Enjoy the successes you achieve and love your child unconditionally.

- Don't become overwhelmed: All ASD kids develop differently and it can be frightening to think of the future. Remember that kids with ASD have a whole lifetime to develop and the more you help, the better the outcome.

Provide structure and safety.

Your child requires routine in order to feel safe in the home but can often struggle to take information from one place to another. If your child uses sign language at school, it does not mean that they will do so at home. Try and keep communication techniques and other behavioral cues consistent.

Create a schedule.

This is another way you can create structure for your child. Meal times should be consistent as should bedtimes. If there is going to be a disruption, then make sure you prepare your child in advance and provide assurance that normality will return.

Positive reinforcement.

Children with ASD need encouragement. Whenever you find a behavior that is worthy of praise then make sure you voice it and be specific about that praise. Stickers and stars are a great way to show your child they have done a good job.

Safety Zone.

Your child will need a safe place they can go when they are overwhelmed with their emotions. Use your knowledge of your kid to make a place that soothes them and makes them feel secure. Lighting and textures will allow them to relax and feel better. This also needs to be private, so your child can be sure they can take their time before they face others.

Nonverbal communication

Communication is a key part of everyday life, but a child with ASD can find traditional methods difficult. If verbal communication is not an option, you need to find another way to connect with your child.

Nonverbal cues will help you understand what your child is trying to tell you. Facial expressions and gesturing will indicate when they are hungry or tired and these actions will often be accompanied by sounds. Taking note of these cues will help other people to understand your child's needs.

Body language and tone of voice will also allow you to communicate with your child successfully. Every gesture you make will mean something to them and just the simplest touch can convey how you feel about them. Your child is communicating with you constantly, even if they never speak a word.

Make time for fun.

A child with ASD is still a child and it can be easy to forget they need fun as well as therapy. Pick a time that your child is at their most alert and plan activities that make your child happy. Do they respond to music and enjoy dancing? Put the stereo on and let yourself bond with your child on the dance floor. Therapy can put a great deal of pressure on a child and it is important to provide light relief.

Make sure these times are pressure free and fun for both of you. The benefits that result from enjoying each other's company can be amazing. Your child is an extraordinary individual and you should revel in that fact.

Sensory sensitivities.

A child with ASD is likely to be hypersensitive to light, sound, smell, and taste and can be affected by the simplest change in the environment. Food preparation can trigger a reaction as the smells can be up to ten times stronger to their senses. All children are different but among the most common offensive smells to ASD children are perfume, shampoo and shower gel, animal smells, body odor, farting, and air freshener.

White noise can also trigger a reaction and your child's hearing will pick out any ambient noise whenever it can.

You may be in a quiet environment, yet your child is having a reaction that you cannot explain.

A quick scan of the room could reveal a fish tank in the room. The noise of the filter could elicit a reaction in a child with ASD.

Understanding your child is a learning curve that you need to embrace. Become the student and tune into your child. Essentially you are learning a new language and the benefits are multiple.

How Do You Like The Book So Far?

ENTER THE LINK BELOW TO LEAVE FEEDBACK ON AMAZON

https://www.amazon.com/review/create-review?asin=B07JL8214P

If you're undecided, just leave a review later...

CHAPTER 3

HOW TO HANDLE THE FOUR MOST CHALLENGING BEHAVIORS OF AUTISM

Every parent and caregiver needs to be responsive and sensitive to children's needs. When you have a child with autism, the level of sensitivity needs to be hyper aware. Your child is using behavior to communicate with you as they are unable to tell you what they need in traditional ways.

You need to be able to translate these behaviors and recognize what your child is telling you. These four behaviors are the most challenging and here we will discuss what they mean and offer advice on how to handle them.

Food Sensitivity

Mealtimes can be a nightmare with autistic children as they are incredibly picky and limited in what they will eat. This is a sensory thing and the best way to find foods that your child will enjoy is by trial and error.

In order to expand their tolerance to food begin by introducing food to the table. It does not necessarily need to progress to the child's plate, but by taking small steps you can raise their tolerance levels gradually.

Your child needs to eat food from the main food groups in order to thrive and grow so the aim is to make sure they are not refusing to eat foods from one or more of these groups. A food diary can help you determine the foods your child enjoys. Autistic children are hyperaware of every aspect of the eating experience and by keeping a diary you can determine the foods and the environment that are the best for your child.

What to include in your food diary.

- What time of the day did they eat? 10.30 am

- What was eaten? Cheese slice

- Who brought the food? Mum

- Which room did they eat it in? Kitchen

- How much was consumed? 4 slices

- Who else was in the room? Mum and sister

- What was the reaction of the other people? Sister praised child and Mum carried on with housework

- Where there any other factors in the environment? The TV was on in the background

All of these factors could affect your child and the way they see food. Some autistic children will only eat food of one color or texture and this can limit their diet. Use imagination to present food in a favorable way and make food a pleasure rather than a cause of stress.

Sleep Disruption

Sleep can be contentious for kids with autism as their nervous system is highly sensitive. This means that even the slightest disruption to their routine can disrupt their sleep for that night.

Limiting the number of stimulants your child has after a certain time in the day will help. Plenty of exercises and mental stimulation will also help to tire out your child.

Be aware of the environmental aspects. Creating a nocturnal oasis for your child will help, a white noise machine, blackout blinds and weighted blankets will all aid sleep. Try having an emergency kit in case your child wakes in the night. Keep a picture of a clock in there with the time they are allowed to get up on it along with a picture of Mom and Dad. Their favorite soft toy or a nightlight can also be included.

Meltdowns

These are going to happen. Fact. The only things you can do are be prepared and recognize how you can minimize the impact.

First, you must realize that when you have a child with autism there are going to be limitations on the social events you can attend. Your child should never be put in a situation that will cause them needless stress and you need to know their limits.

Recognize the difference between a tantrum and a meltdown. With a tantrum, the child is in control and are merely using their anger to get their own way. A meltdown is completely different. Your child no longer has control and as they are overwhelmed with their emotions. They are unable to calm down using traditional methods and you need to ride out the storm in the safest way possible. Soothe your child by holding them and keeping them safe until the meltdown has passed.

As with tantrums when a meltdown occurs in public it can lead to unwanted attention from the public. Hurtful comments and reactions can be curtailed by simply having wallet size cards on hand to give out to strangers. "My child is autistic, please visit these websites to learn more" followed by a list of helpful sites can help public awareness of autism. These can be obtained from autism societies or you can make your own.

Aggression

Autistic children will often use aggressive behavior and self-injury to express their frustration. Understanding why your child is so frustrated will help you minimize this behavior and support their needs. As with the food diary, take notes about when the aggressive behavior occurs.

Make a note of food intake, length of sleep and other environmental factors. Are there times when one caregiver is absent, and this leads to an increase in aggression? Be aware that even seasons can affect your child. Barometric pressure can cause pain with sinuses and extreme cold similarly affects your child's comfort.

How should you deal with this aggressive behavior? All children will respond differently, but a general rule of thumb is to follow these steps.

- Consider safety first and move any objects that can cause harm

- Take yourself out of your child's zone

- Speak loudly and clearly using single words. "Stop" "No" and "Behave" will let them know that what they are doing is unacceptable.

- Allow them time to cool off after their behavior has stopped..

CHAPTER 4

EXERCISES FOR AUTISTIC CHILDREN

For children with autism, it is important to engage in vigorous activities for at least an hour a day to promote overall health. Increased exercise also helps decrease hyperactivity and aggression. Not all exercises are ideal for autistic kids, but these five will help your child increase coordination, endurance, and strength in your child.

Important tip: When teaching your autistic child a new exercise it is important to do so in a calm and laid-back manner. Verbal cues can encourage your child to progress and using your hands to guide them through movements will reduce the chance of frustration and upset.

Tips before beginning an exercise program

- Consult your health expert before any new exercises for a child with autism

- Begin slowly and monitor your child for signs of fatigue. If you push your child beyond their comfort zone it will be difficult to encourage them to repeat the experience. Be aware of shortness of breath and muscle cramps and stop whenever you see signs of either.

- Be prepared. Make sure the child is well rested and fully hydrated before beginning any vigorous activity. Make sure you have water readily available to hydrate during the session.

Mirror Exercises

Autism is classically marked by inability to interact with others and lack of social skills. This exercise will not only improve coordination and body strength but is an ideal way to improve social interaction and body awareness.

- Stand facing your child with your hands resting at you side.

- Begin moving your arms in circles and encourage your child to mirror these movements. Increase the speed and complexity of your movements at regular intervals.

- While you are both making the arm movements try touching fingertips for added interaction.

- Incorporate your head and legs in the movement and encourage your child to initiate other cycles.

- Continue this activity for five minutes and then rest. Repeat up to five times.

Star Jumps

Exercises that involve jumping are great full body exercises that aid cardiovascular improvement. They also help improve core strength and development of legs and calves. Star jumps are perfect as they can be performed anywhere and are great fun!

- Begin in a squatting position as close to the ground as possible. Tuck arms into the chest and make sure feet are flat to the floor

- Launch from the floor extending arms and legs to create a cross effect.

- When you land resume the squatting stance and repeat the action until fatigued.

Grab Ball Complex

Stand opposite your child using markers to aid special awareness while you hold a ball in your hands.

Move the ball in various positions and encourage your child to reach out and touch the ball. Begin with movements that are close to your body until your child is comfortable with the ball and then progress. Move the ball in a way that will encourage the child to bend and rotate as far as possible and create sequences that they can follow.

Scramble

The scramble is a great warm up activity that can be adapted to include other movements to suit your child. These are the basic premise you can use to build your own scramble.

- Lie flat on a soft surface, a yoga mat is perfect.

- Raise to quadruped position, with knees and hands on the floor.

- Stand quickly with bent knees and jump into the air

Use verbal cues to teach your child to return to specific positions. For instance, a single clap can mean a return to lying position while two claps mean hands and knees. Adding other positions will increase their listening skills and help them discriminate between positions.

Medicine Ball Slams

Throwing heavy objects not only increases physical strength and coordination but it can also have other therapeutic benefits. Slamming heavy objects can help relieve frustration and stimulates the brain center.

- Stand tall and hold the medicine ball with both hands.

- Raise the ball overhead still holding on with both hands and straight arms.

- Throw the ball to the floor with as much force as possible, maybe accompanied with a grunt.

- Bend carefully at the knees and resume your first position.

- Repeat until fatigued.

This exercise can be made more challenging by introducing a target to aim the ball at or increasing the weight of the ball.

Bear Crawls

This exercise is a great way to improve strength in the trunk and upper body while also developing coordination and motor skills.

- Begin by kneeling on the floor on all fours, hands directly under the shoulder area and knees under hips.

- Spread legs out to the rear and splay the fingers to increase contact with the floor.

- Walk in this position for a short distance, maybe fifteen feet at the first try.

- Keeping this position track back along the way you have just come.

- Once this move has been mastered switch up the speed and directions to achieve optimal results.

- Encourage your child by helping them raise their hips if needed.

Compound exercises and all body exercises are perfect for autistic children to use several muscle groups at the same time. Check your area for groups that encourage exercise for children and when you feel your child is ready maybe join them for a session. Meet with the organizers beforehand and explain the difficulties your child encounters with their autism.

Shared activities can help your child develop their social skills as well as their physical development. Sharing information with the organizers and other children that attend will make the situation more comfortable for everyone involved.

CHAPTER 5

WHAT HELP IS AVAILABLE FOR CAREGIVERS?

Caring for a child with ASD requires energy and time. Parenting is a stressful role but even more so when your child has special needs. Don't try to do everything on your own, make use of the help and assistance available to you. If you need a helping hand, support and even financial support here are a few places you can turn to.

ADS support groups

Joining these groups can help you feel less alone in the world. Sharing information, support and experiences will help you cope with the reality of raising a child with autism. There is a wealth of groups out there, some for parents and others for caregivers that are filled with nuggets of wisdom. Facebook groups can help you share your experiences and pass on tips and assure you that you are not alone.

Respite Care

Every parent needs a break, and this is especially true for parents of ASD children. The National Autistic Service provides a short break service that allows both adults and children to take time out from their home life. Use the contacts in your groups to arrange respite breaks for yourself and your child. Everybody benefits from time away from a stressful situation.

External help

As a prime caregiver, you need to know your child's rights when applying for help from the government. The federal law known as the Individuals with Disabilities Education Act ensures that children with ASD are eligible for low cost or free treatments.

These include speech and physical therapy, psychological services, and other specialized treatments.

It is important to know that these treatments are available to infants under ten without an official diagnosis. If your child is developing at a slower rate than other children, you are eligible for help.

There are two stages to the help you can apply for depending on the age of your child.

Services for Early Intervention

Children up to the age of two years old can receive help through this service. They will need to undergo a free evaluation to assess their rate of development. If the service indicates that help is required, you will work with specialists to develop a program that will help your child increase development rates.

For an autistic child, this program will include therapies to aid speech and physical development and also the importance of playing. The aim of these intervention services is to help your child prepare for a school environment and interaction with other children. The therapies can be conducted in a care center or in a domestic setting.

Autism source is a helpful site that will tell you how to get a referral for this service or you can ask your pediatrician.

Special Education Service

Children over the age of three will be encouraged to receive help from programs that are based in schools. The goal of the program is to find the least restrictive environment suitable for their individual needs. Every child is different and will require individual help, but this program strives to place a child in a "normal" classroom for at least part of the day. Your local school will conduct an evaluation of your child and this will determine the program they will follow. An education plan will be drawn up that will clearly state the educational goals for the next twelve months and the support the school will provide.

Sometimes parents can feel the care of their child is being managed by others and can feel left out. This should never be the case, you are the voice of your child and as such should know your rights.

Parents of children with ASD have a legal right to the following

- Involvement in any plan or treatment course developed for your Child, this applies from the beginning of treatment and continues throughout.

- You have the legal right to disagree with any decisions made by the school system. Nobody knows your child's needs better than you do.

- You may seek an evaluation from outside the system.

- The education plan for your child will be managed by a team. You have the legal right to invite whoever you want to join the team. This could be a relative or a medical expert, you can ask any number of people to be the voice of your child.

- You can ask for a meeting of the team at any time you need. Providing you allow for the needs of everyone involved you can address any issues you have with your child's development.

- If all else fails and you cannot agree with the school and/or the team you can seek legal help. This will be provided for free or at a low price depending on your circumstances.

Computer programs and apps for autistic children.

Advances in technology have provided an abundance of tools for educating autistic children. IPads have become an essential tool to help learners with autism and it is worth checking out the following programs.

Jacob's Lessons: Created by a father to create a fun and interactive app to use with his young daughter. The site helps learners to develop skills in gender recognition, object functionality and object recognition. The user is encouraged with both verbal and visual cues when they provide a correct answer.

Model Me Kids: Narration and graphics are used to teach the finer points of social skills. By breaking down activities into small steps an autistic child can learn at a pace that suits them.

Vizzle: This is an innovative program that provides support and for parents and educators of children with ASD.

CONCLUSION

Now you have the information you need to help you on your journey. Your child is incredibly special, and you will have an amazing time together learning from each other. Enjoy your time together and share your experiences with others. Autism is misunderstood by many people and part of your remit as a parent is to make more people aware and allow autistic children more freedom. Stop those negative reactions by explaining your child's behavior and sharing information.

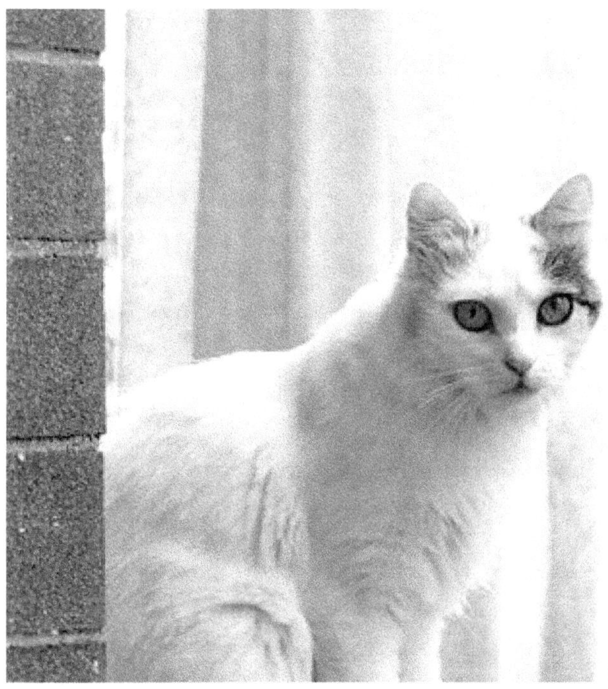

And finally, if you liked the book, I would like to ask you to do me a favor and leave a review for the book on Amazon. Just go to your account on Amazon or enter the link below.

ENETR THE LINK BELOW TO LEAVE A REVIEWS ON AMAZON!
https://www.amazon.com/review/create-review?asin=B07JL8214P

Thank you and good luck!

ACKNOWLEDGEMENTS

https://www.helpguide.com

https://www.healthline.com

https://www.babble.com

https://www.todaysparent.com